TABLE OF CONTENTS

PRESENTATION

39% of adults aged 18 years and over were overweight in 2014, and 13% were obese. They found that most of the world's population live in countries where overweight and obesity kills more people than underweight. These numbers describe a tragic public health situation. Being overweight increases a person's risk of serious illness. A very large (and growing) percentage of citizens are at increased risk for developing serious chronic diseases, and face the prospect of early disability or death as the result of being overweight. Meanwhile the entire society struggles under the burden of the resulting increase in health care costs. This book concerns weight loss, an issue constantly on many people's minds. Most everyone wants to be slim and toned, but the reality is that it is far easier to gain weight than to lose it. On the following pages causes of weight gain are reviewed, along with numerous reasons why people should devote the effort necessary to reduce their weight to recommended levels. Having provided motivation for a weight loss program, we conclude with a discussion of weight loss methods, and suggestions for achieving permanent healthy weight loss

You may have been spreading honey on your toast for a few years, but people have been using it to treat illnesses for thousands of years! Now honey is being used to make a product that can help wounds heal more quickly.

BEING OVERWEIGHT

Being overweight or clinically obese is when you have a high calorie intake and low energy expenditure. To lose weight, you can either reduce your calorie intake, or do regular exercise and reduce calorie intake at the same time. Doing exercise too is always more beneficial. Many people don't exercise correctly when they want to lose weight. They think if they do a high-impact cardio workout or work out for very long periods of time, they'll lose weight quicker and keep it off. But actually it's not effective this way. It's important not to exert too much stress on the body, as you would actually be losing the benefit of the workout overall. It's therefore important to choose activities on a daily basis that are not going to put unnecessary stress on the body.

GRADUAL AND REGULAR EXERCISE

Gradual, regular physical activity and healthy diet is crucial for losing weight, keeping it off and maintaining a healthy lifestyle. A well-balanced programme of exercises must include both strength exercises and aerobic exercises. Strength exercises are important for increasing muscle mass, as it's the muscles that burn the most calories from your diet. Aerobic activities such as walking, running, swimming, cycling, and in general all the activities that use large muscle groups are great for losing weight and toning up.

Regular physical activity reduces the risk of cardiovascular disease, diabetes, high blood pressure and being obese and can actually help you to look and feel younger for longer.

THE RIGHT AMOUNT OF EXERCISE IS IMPORTANT

In extreme cases, excess physical activity can have negative effects on weight loss. Under normal conditions, cortisol – known as the stress hormone acts to help the body overcome stressful situations such as prolonged fasting. Higher and more prolonged levels of cortisol in the bloodstream have been shown to have negative effects on the body and actually deposit fat especially the abdomen.

EXERCISING ON AN EMPTY STOMACH

It's common for dieters to lose weight by exercising on an empty stomach. It does have its advantages, but can also be risky to your health. The recommended duration of aerobic exercise on an empty stomach is about 40 minutes; over this period and you may be at risk of using protein as your energy supply resulting in muscle catabolism – the destruction of muscle mass.

BURN CALORIES EVEN WHEN YOU'RE RESTING

It's natural to reduce the amount you eat to reduce calorie intake. But by adopting drastic measures, such as diets based only on eating fruits and vegetables or eliminating certain foods altogether will only result in a loss of weight due to fluid loss and muscle mass.

This is not achievable or healthy to maintain over a long period of time. Just by moving, you're burning calories therefore muscle mass needs to be maintained because muscles have a high basal metabolic rate (BMR) and this affects the rate you burn calories and ultimately whether you maintain, gain, or lose weight. Your basal metabolic rate accounts for about 60 to 75% of the calories you burn every day. Physical activity and nutrition are two complementary elements. If you want to lose weight in a smart way, you need to combine the right amount of physical activity with the right diet.

Often people who want to achieve their weight goal adopt restrictive and drastic diets to get immediate results. Diets that are about losing weight fast are actually very harmful to your health.

STEADY PHYSICAL ACTIVITY IS IMPORTANT

To lose weight effectively and safely you need to be patient and follow a healthy and balanced diet, coupled with a programme of steady physical activity; increasing in duration. This way, you'll lose weight but not your health. And to get good results in the long term, you should also get advice from a doctor, a nutritionist or a dietician who will recommend the right diet; taking into account the right calorie intake depending on the exercise programme you want to do and your specific goals.

DAILY PHYSICAL ACTIVITY

In order to benefit from exercising, you have to gradually increase the intensity and frequency of training. This is key for overall weight loss. Physical activity should be done every day or at least five times a week. To lose weight, it's ideal to train for 6-7 days a week for 40-50 minutes, rather than train three times a week for two hours. Even just 30 minutes of daily physical exercises broken into three sessions of 10 minutes every day may be sufficient to increase your basal metabolic rate (BMR).

WHAT THE BASAL METABOLIC RATE IS

The basal metabolic rate affects the rate that you burn calories and ultimately whether you maintain, gain, or lose weight. Your basal metabolic rate accounts for about 60 to 75% of the calories you burn every day. When you start exercising, you consume more or less in equal parts carbohydrates and lipids, especially if you work at a low intensity and for a limited time. After about an hour of activity up to 80% of lipids are required for energy, and only 20% of glucose and / or glycogen. As the intensity of exercise increases - the use of fatty acids and glucose increases. Therefore physical activity and nutrition are two complementary elements.

NUTRITION FOR EFFECTIVE WEIGHT LOSS

The easiest solution might be to eat less, eliminating some particular foods from your diet, but this actually limits the supply of nutrients essential for the body. The goal is to consume more calories but reduce your calorie intake by limiting (not eliminating) foods that contain too many calories and empty calories. If you do aerobic activity long-term, you'll need large quantities of carbohydrates to avoid energy crash due to lack of sugar. If you're more of a body builder, you'll require high amounts of protein. By reducing the intake of protein weight loss occurs at the expense of muscle mass and proteins that make up the organs such as the heart and kidneys. Diets low in carbohydrates and rich in protein instead can be harmful especially for bones, kidneys and cholesterol. All diets based on the consumption of large amounts of certain foods are harmful not only physically, but also psychologically. Your body needs energy to perform

The correct amount of nutrients (carbohydrates, proteins, fats, water, vitamins and minerals) will vary according to the individual's lifestyle. Carbohydrates should cover about 60% of your needs, the remainder being 25% fat and 15% protein. The time between eating and starting physical activity, can greatly improve performance. It is recommended, before exercise, to eat a meal consisting of carbohydrates. While carbohydrate-containing foods such as yogurt, fruit and cereal takes one to two hours to be digested, foods high in fat will take more than four hours and is not ideal. Maintain a steady diet and physical activity that reduces body fat without affecting lean muscle mass.

TRAINING ON AN EMPTY STOMACH

Training on an empty stomach can increase the risk of seizures from lack of sugar, characterised by sweating, a feeling of faintness, paleness and dizziness. If you feel like this, eat foods immediately that contain a lot of sugar like chocolate, honey or sugary drinks, or even better eat a meal rich in carbohydrates. Trying to lose weight through diet alone can be very restrictive, not always effective and difficult to maintain over a long period of time. It's better to mix a healthy balanced diet with physical activity.

Main things to remember:

- Be patient. Do not be in a hurry to lose weight
- Eat a bit of everything in moderation
- Have five small meals a day: your metabolism is maintained by eating moderately several times a day rather than over-eating during mealtimes. A snack mid-morning and mid-afternoon leads to eating a little less for lunch or dinner
- Drink at least two litres of water a day for proper bodily hydration
- Do regular physical activities even for just 30 minutes a day
- Don't forget to also relax and get some rest.

Being overweight increases your risk of long-term health problems that could shorten your life, like diabetes and cardiovascular disease. Preventing these serious illnesses is often the main health reason for losing weight.

REDUCE YOUR RISK OF DISEASE

Reducing your risk of serious life-threatening illnesses is an important health benefit. Many people may feel that the best reward for losing weight is feeling healthier and seeing an improvement. One of things you might notice is having more energy and an increase in your fitness.

Just 30 minutes a day

Even just 30 minutes of daily physical exercises broken into three sessions of 10 minutes of physical activity every day may be sufficient to increase the basal metabolic rate (BMR) and this affects the rate that you burn calories and ultimately whether you maintain, gain, or lose weight.

Your basal metabolic rate accounts for about 60 to 75% of the calories you burn every day. To feel the benefits of exercising, you have to gradually increase the intensity and frequency of training. This is key for overall weight loss. So you should do physical activity every day or at least five times a week.

THE IMPORTANCE OF BODY MASS INDEX (BMI)

In general, body composition is divided into fat mass, and lean mass and can be measured by height, weight, circumferences and skinfold thickness. Two approaches are commonly used to determine if people are overweight: the body mass index (BMI) and waist measurement. The BMI helps to determine how much you weigh in relation to your height. Waist measurements give you an idea of how fat is distributed in your body. The BMI is the most common way to try to work out if you're overweight or very overweight (obese). It measures the relationship between weight and height. People who have a BMI over 30 are considered to be obese. Being obese is a greater risk to health than being overweight. People who have a BMI between 25 and 30 are usually considered to be overweight. Being overweight alone does not necessarily cause health problems, but it could be a problem if the person already has certain illnesses, such as type 2 diabetes. Although useful and simple to calculate, BMI doesn't take into account the physique and muscle mass of the person.

PREDICTING RISK OF OBESITY

Measuring the circumference of the body is more accurate for predicting the risk of obesity. The distribution of body fat is an important predictor of the risk of obesity. The circumference of the arm, waist, hips, thigh is taken into account to obtain an estimate of body composition. You can get a better idea of how fat is distributed in your body by looking at the relationship between your waist and your hips. If you have a relatively big amount of belly fat, your risk of disease is higher. The waist / hip ratio, waist / thigh, waist circumference or neck measurements provide information on the level of risk of hypertension, metabolic syndrome, type 2 diabetes, dyslipidemia, coronary artery disorders and premature death.

The overall benefits of losing weight:

• An increase in lean body mass and reduction in fat mass

• An increase in the efficiency of the use of fats and carbohydrates in food

• An increased metabolism and energy expenditure even while resting

• An improvement in cardiovascular efficiency

• Lower blood pressure

• A reduction in the risk of developing cardiovascular problems and metabolic diseases

• A reduction in LDL cholesterol (harmful cholesterol), triglycerides and fat accumulated and deposited on a visceral level.

If you do regular physical activity, it will be easier for you to lose weight than people who have a more sedentary lifestyle. To really benefit from losing weight, a complete physical activity programme must include both strength and aerobic exercises to increase muscles and tone the body, as muscles are important to burn off calories and promote weight loss.

From understanding what metabolism means and how it can help with weight loss to finding out if exercising on an empty stomach is really a good thing – discover all the answers to your questions.

WHAT IS METABOLISM

Metabolism can be defined as the speed at which the body burns calories to meet the energy demands of the body. Metabolism is the process by which your body converts what you eat and drink into energy. During this complex biochemical process, calories in food and drinks are combined with oxygen to release the energy your body needs to function.

WHICH FACTORS INFLUENCE METABOLISM?

Metabolism is influenced by physical activity, diet and the basal metabolic rate (BMR). BMR is the energy needed in rest conditions to maintain vital functions such as breathing, your heart beating and your organs working. In someone with a sedentary lifestyle, the BMR will be less than that of someone who's physically active. Physical activity can increase energy expenditure at rest because a greater amount of muscle mass has greater metabolic demands therefore they use up more calories.

HOW DO YOU SPEED UP METABOLISM?

It is recommended that mixed activity which consists of high intensity exercises, toning with weights or machines and aerobic activity such as running, swimming, as well as walking and cycling. This promotes an increase in muscle mass with an increase in metabolism even during rest and a reduction of fat mass. Good muscle tone helps to burn more calories both during exercise and after it. Strength and endurance exercises also maintain a high energy expenditure for several hours after the end of the training session.

WHAT IS THE CORRECT WORKOUT INTENSITY FOR WEIGHT LOSS?

The ideal intensity of physical activity for weight loss is by exercising with a workload and maintaining a heart rate of 60-70% compared to the maximum one. Knowing your Maximum Heart Rate (MHR) allows you to set more accurate heart rate training zones for the highest level of effectiveness, enjoyment and weight loss. It can also show improvement over time, giving you critical feedback on your fitness level.

HOW DO YOU WORK OUT THE MHR?

The MHR can be calculated different ways. The simplest way is to subtract your age from 220. 85% Intensity: (220 − (age = 40)) × 0.85 → 153 bpm. The Karvonen method factors in resting heart rate (HRrest) to calculate target heart rate (THR), using a range of 50–85% intensity: THR = ((HRmax − HRrest) × % intensity) + HR. This will give you the value frequency to maintain during exercise in order to burn fat and lose weight.

IS IT EFFECTIVE EXERCISING ON AN EMPTY STOMACH?

Exercising on an empty stomach definitely has advantages because it increases the use of lipids due to the reduced blood sugar level that you have in the morning. It's ideal not to do too much exercise on an empty stomach – anything up to about 30 minutes doesn't pose a threat to your health, but longer than this can cause muscle catabolism, where the muscle proteins are used to obtain energy resulting in muscle shrinkage.

IT IS BEST TO WORK WITH WEIGHTS BEFORE DOING AEROBIC EXERCISES?

It depends on the person and their specific weight goal. Generally it's ideal to do some weights first in strength training to use up carbohydrates and then do some aerobic exercises.

WHAT IS THE RIGHT AMOUNT OF NUTRIENTS FOR MODERATE ACTIVITY?

The energy derived from the three major macro-nutrients – carbohydrates, fats and proteins varies according to your lifestyle. To cover energy needs, you must have the correct amount of nutrients (carbohydrates, proteins, fats, water, vitamins and minerals). Carbohydrates should cover about 60% of individual needs, the remainder being 25% fat and 15% protein.

HOW TO LOSE WEIGHT

The best way for you to lose weight fast will depend on your starting point, your end goal, and your lifestyle. In this article we lay out ten strategies that are applicable to everyone, whether you're a fitness novice looking to shed several stone, or you simply require motivation to keep going. Generally speaking the best way to lose weight quickly, and maintain that weight loss, is to follow a steady, manageable plan. Don't try to take on more than you can reasonably fit into one day, unless you're willing to make the sacrifice. Most likely sleep or your social life.

The NHS recommends that you aim to lose no more than 2 lbs (1kg) per week; anymore than that and you risk burning out and giving up. With that in mind, here are ten strategies to get you losing weight quickly.

1. ACHIEVE A CONSISTENT CALORIE DEFICIT

The short answer to the question of how to lose weight fast is to achieve a consistent calorie deficit. That is, burn more calories than you consume. If you eat 2,500 calories a day – the recommended daily amount for a man, although of course this can vary wildly depending on your height, weight and frame – and burn 3,000, you are in a calorie deficit. If, however, you burn 3,000 but have consumed 3,500, you're not in a calorie deficit, even though you've almost certainly been working out a lot have burned that much energy. What you need to do is ensure you're eating the right food and doing the right exercise so that you're sufficiently full and satisfied even when consuming fewer calories than you burn. Here's how...

2. DECREASE CALORIE INPUT THROUGH DIET CHANGES

As we alluded to above, a common pitfall that many people experience when trying to lose weight is that as they start exercising more, they feel like they need to eat more to keep their energy levels up and consequently fail to see results. Instead, we recommend adapting your diet to get the most out of your calories. All foods have different energy densities. Foods like fruits, vegetables and whole grains have low energy density, which means you will get fuller faster when eating these than you would high energy density foods. Proteins and healthy fats promote more stable blood glucose levels, keeping you fuller across a time period and less likely to crave sugar or over eat, and so these are the kinds of foods you should get the majority of your calories from. Consuming the same amount of calories as you are now (or fewer if possible), but getting more nutritional value from them will help you feel fuller for longer and lose weight more quickly as a result.

3. DON'T CUT OUT ALL OF ANY SINGLE FOOD GROUP

We all know that some foods – and some food groups – are healthier than others, and that we need every type of food in our diet. The problem is that many of us aren't getting the right balance. The best way to reduce weight and maintain the weight loss is by simply eating a balanced and healthy diet, without refusing yourself particular foods... If you do cut out foods, you need to make sure your diet is still balanced and you are getting the nutrients your body needs from other sources." For example, unless you're training to become a weightlifter, there's nothing wrong with carbs per se – despite what keto diet fans might tell you – but the biggest food culprit when it comes to hindering weight loss is the simple carbohydrate. Could complete meal replacement product Huel help you diet effectively? Compared to complex carbs like beans, whole grains and vegetables, which break down and release energy slowly, thereby keeping you full and energised, simple carbs such as sugar and starchy foods which break down into sugars – such as pasta and spuds – give you a shorter boost of energy, then leave you wanting more.

The likelihood is that the more simple carbs you eat, the more you'll end up eating overall, harming the balance of your calorie deficit. One easy trick if you're a carb fan is to swap out white pasta or rice for courgetti, or noodles made from other vegetables like butternut squash. This can make an arrabiata, curry or stir fry much lower in calories. You'll hardly notice the difference when you're eating it, but you'll be fuller for longer despite consuming fewer calories.

4. TRY A FOOD SUBSTITUTE

Sometimes it's a real struggle to reduce the calories you take in, or even just to track them. If you're constantly on the move and don't have the time to count calories, or you have the best intentions and are cooking fresh with ingredients that aren't all labeled with their nutrition info broken down, then accurately tracking calories can be a nightmare.

To ensure you're getting a good mix of nutrients, as well as all-important protein. This is not marketed as a dietary aid, but it is highly nutritious, and makes calorie counting a lot easier.

5. TRY INTERMITTENT FASTING

Some people thrive on intermittent fasting, which means significantly cutting calories – or completely fasting – for a portion of the day or week, and then eating normally for the rest. The most popular form of intermittent fasting is the 5:2 diet, where you eat normally for five days a week but then eating no more than 600 calories two days a week. There's also the 16:8 diet, which is a bit different. With this diet you can eat anything for 8 hours a day, but can only drink water during a 16 hour fast. The recommended time to eat is between 10am and 6pm, although this can be flexible depending on what time you'd prefer to start or end eating (as long as you stay within an eight hour window).

The benefits of intermittent fasting is that during the fast period the body will run out of carbohydrates to run on, and so start to take energy from the body's fat stores, thus starting to burn that belly fat once and for all.

6. DRINK MORE WATER AND LESS ALCOHOL

Drinking more water – especially before a meal – can help us to feel fuller, thereby helping us to stop eating sooner and consume fewer calories than we otherwise would have. What's more, few of us consider what we drink when we total up our daily calorie count and so potentially hundreds of extra calories can sneak into our bodies. Replacing fruit juices, fizzy drinks and even tea and coffee with water means we can save up our calorie allowance for the good stuff: the food that fills us up. Top tip: keep a reusable water bottle with you at all times and restrict what else you drink. This can feel like a hard habit to break at first, but is surprisingly easy to maintain once you have a zero calorie drink to hand 24/7. Reducing the amount of alcohol we drink also comes with benefits. Most obviously, alcoholic drinks are often very calorific, so drinking less alcohol means consuming fewer calories. Simple. Secondly, drinking alcohol increases our appetite, so we're more likely to eat more than usual – and more of the bad stuff – when we've been drinking. Cheesy chips, I'm looking at you. Lastly, we all know how we feel after a night of heavy drinking. Ready for a session and the gym and a day eating fruit, veg and simple carbohydrates? We didn't think so. Drinking alcohol not only means we take in more calories at the time, but can affect our ability to function well and make healthy choices the next day.

7. INCREASE CALORIE OUTPUT THROUGH EXERCISE

Now we've tackled diet and nutrition (calories in), it's time to look at exercise (calories out). Even if you're eating healthily and are reasonably active in your daily life, it's unlikely you'll be able to lose weight quickly without additional exercise, whether that's running, gym, crossfit, team sports, cycling or any of the other myriad activities available. What's more, working out will make you look and feel better and in our view, once you start looking and feeling better, it gets a lot easier to find the will power needed to improve your diet. When it comes to choosing what type of exercise you do, the most important thing is that it's something you enjoy and will stick to. Don't force yourself to run if chances are you'll be walking ten minutes in.

8. FOCUS ON WEIGHT TRAINING IN ADDITION TO CARDIO

There are two main types of exercise: cardio training and weight – or resistance –training. Both burn calories, the difference is that whilst cardio burns a lot of calories upfront, weight training continues to to burn calories post workout. This is because weight training builds muscle, and muscle burns more than fat as you carry out day-to-day tasks. In short, the greater your muscle:fat ratio, the more calories you burn even when you are standing still. Weight training may seem daunting, but you don't have to join a gym and face up to the squat rack right away. There are so many weight exercises you can do at home with simple bits of equipment from dumbbells to kettlebells, and balls to ropes.

9. VARY THE INTENSITY OF YOUR WORKOUTS

As well doing both cardio and weight training, if you want to lose weight it's also important to vary the intensity with which you exercise. In any given week, and within any given workout, you should exercise both aerobically (a little out of breath but not gasping) and anaerobically (going flat out, like when running for a bus). Aerobic exercise needs oxygen to give muscles energy and generally requires moderate exertion. Examples include gentler running, cycling and swimming.

It's a crucial part of losing weight quickly because it uses both sugar and fat as its energy source, but to burn fat you need to do it for long enough that you've burned through your sugar stores first. Anaerobic exercise, on the other hand, primarily uses sugar as its fuel. This doesn't mean that it's not good for weight loss, though. Anaerobic exercise helps build muscle, and as we explained above, this will help you burn calories even when you're resting. Anaerobic exercises are generally high intensity, for example sprinting and weight lifting. A running watch or fitness tracker will help you to know what intensity exercise you're doing. As they either have built-in heart-rate trackers or pair with ones you strap to your chest, they can show you how hard you're working out and let you know when you need to push it harder.

10. TRACK YOUR INPUT VS. OUTPUT (THAT ALL IMPORTANT CALORIE DEFICIT)

It's important to decide how you want to measure your success and track consistently, understand that you will see daily fluctuations due to things like digestive contents and water retention. Running watches are the easiest way to track your progress, remain motivated and keep weight off. Depending how fancy you go, you can track pretty much any metric that works for you, certainly way beyond whether you've achieved your 10,000 steps. Whether it's weight, BMI, resting heart rate, calories burned or activity level, the best running watch will track it all. Many wearables branded as fitness trackers also have a stab at these more advanced metrics nowadays, but we'd always recommend a watch over a band. Another way to keep track of your progress is the old fashioned method of weighing yourself. The great thing about modern bathroom scales is they don't just tell you your weight; they also let you know your body fat percentage.

WAY TO LOSE WEIGHT FOR MEN

Dropping over 3 pounds of our body weight is not that easy attributing to our unhealthy lifestyles. Most of us tend to lead sedentary lifestyles leaving every work to machines. Well, however hard it may seem, this is actually an achievable goal. You only need a healthy diet accompanied by regular exercise, and you are there.

THE FASTEST WAY TO LOSE WEIGHT

If you can burn 500 calories above what you consume per week, it is likely that you will be shedding between 1 and 2 pounds of your overall weight. The idea here is for you to ensure that you eat less and exercising regularly. Keeping off junk food is yet another great way that will ensure you lose weight fast. Point to note – By eating between 1,050 and 1,200 calories daily and keeping to the gym regularly for at least an hour, you will definitely achieve faster weight loss results. You will start realizing results merely a week after commencing on your weight loss regime. Incorporating top diet pills is also good.

HERE ARE SOME TRICKS TO HELP YOU SHED MORE WEIGHT FASTER

1. **Start your day with a lot of proteins Eggs**

And keep it that way all day. The most important part of losing weight is to cut back on sugars and starches (carbs). They are proven to stimulate secretion of insulin, the main fat storage hormone in our body. In opposition to carbs, proteins can boost metabolism and increase fat burning. Proteins also keep you fuller longer, by reducing your level of the hunger hormone ghrelin.

Here are some delicious high protein breakfast ideas:

• homemade muesli blend with rich in proteins chia seeds, nuts and unsweetened yogurt (no colored yogurt if you want to lose weight!)

• omelet, scrambled eggs and other variation of eggs

• dark bread with unsweetened peanut butter, cottage cheese and avocado

2. Drink sufficient water

Keeping hydrated is very important if you want to stay healthy. The funny thing is that if you drink less water, the body will tend to retain the water weight instead. Yes, every individual differs from another; however, it is recommended that you drink at least 8 glasses (64 ounces) of water daily. Taking water a few minutes to meals helps to reduce the amount of food one is likely to consume considering that it fills up space in the stomach. Plus you are less likely to confuse hunger with thirst.

3. Avoid too much salt

As mentioned earlier, salt triggers weight gain and that is why most us find it hard to bring the scale down. Statistics indicate that salt consumption for an average American is two times the recommended daily consumption. This explains the high number of overweight individuals in America attributing to bloating and the incapability to shed the stubborn fats. Salt makes one feel thirsty and hungrier; hence, make sure you read labels before settling for your package and always go for fresh rather than packaged diets.

4. Check your eating speed

People who eat faster tend to grow fatter than those who take their time (The University of Rhode Island). The body needs up to 20 minutes to communicate to the brain that it has had enough. In this case, if you eat faster, the chances are that satiation signals will elude your fullness feelings and eventually lead to your overeating. Always chew your food properly and be conscious of the fullness signals.

5. Eat more fresh fruits and vegetables

Fresh vegetables and fruits have immense healthy benefits in the body. They can be considered as good source of high fiber diet that helps to keep you full. Taking vegetable soup before meals could help lower the amount of calories consumed by 20%. Thus, if you want to lose weight faster, start with vegetable soup or a small salad before embarking on your main meal.

6. Stay away from junky diets

Well, it is sometimes very hard to stop craving for those junky diets, but you can still manage it. Though it may look very obvious, how we breathe can help in this course. Taking a deep breath can help get you out of that brief stress, improve oxygen circulation in your brain and body tissues and cause a reduction in. It is, therefore, advisable for you to have a few breathing breaks all day. Incorporating walking in the breathe breaks can also help to take away stress. Take a few minutes strolling in silence; a few deep breathes and results will start to show up. Yoga is also one better way of managing your cravings.

7. Check your emotions

Men tend to neglect their emotional state and focus most on their calorie consumption and hence, end up gaining weight instead. Your emotional condition significantly reflects in your health and overall being. Your feelings prior to meals – hungry, bored or sad – are likely to impact on your weight loss achievement. To succeed in your weight lose endeavours, working hard and staying focused is mandatory. The best way to do so is by recording whatever you eat and watching over your mood.

WHAT IS HONEY

Honey is a supersaturated solution of sugar made by bees. Honeybees (Apis mellifera) collect a liquid secretion from flowers, called nectar, and take this back to their hives. At the hive, honeybees add enzymes to the nectar, and place it in wax cells where it ripens to form honey. During ripening, the enzymes convert sucrose (a type of sugar in the nectar) into glucose and fructose (other types of sugars).

A thick, golden liquid produced by industrious bees, honey is made using the nectar of flowering plants and is saved inside the beehive for eating during times of scarcity. But how do bees make honey?

Nectar — a sugary liquid is extracted from flowers using a bee's long, tube-shaped tongue and stored in its extra stomach, or "crop." While sloshing around in the crop, the nectar mixes with enzymes that transform its chemical composition and pH, making it more suitable for long-term storage.

When a honeybee returns to the hive, it passes the nectar to another bee by regurgitating the liquid into the other bee's mouth. This regurgitation process is repeated until the partially digested nectar is finally deposited into a honeycomb. Once in the comb, nectar is still a viscous liquid — nothing like the thick honey you use at the breakfast table. To get all that extra water out of their honey, bees set to work fanning the honeycomb with their wings in an effort to speed up the process of evaporation. When most of the water has evaporated from the honeycomb, the bee seals the comb with a secretion of liquid from its abdomen, which eventually hardens into beeswax. Away from air and water, honey can be stored indefinitely, providing bees with the perfect food source for cold winter months.

TYPES OF HONEY

The market currently is flooded with a vast variety of Honey, with each one bearing its characteristic taste, flavor and color. To be precise, there are more than 300 types of honey that exist today and with each one boasting of special set of health and nutritional benefits, Honey lovers are in for a sweet time. While it is hard to evade the temptation of buying a factory made and beautifully packaged bottle of Honey, but if health, purity and quality is what you seek; opt for either of the below given varieties of Honey. Doing so will ensure you the best in taste, flavor and health benefits like no other!

- Acacia Honey
- Alfalfa Honey
- Aster Honey
- Avocado Honey
- Basswood Honey
- Beechwood Honey
- Blueberry Honey
- Bluegum Honey
- Buckwheat Honey
- Clover Honey
- Dandelion Honey
- Eucalyptus Honey
- Fireweed Honey
- Heather Honey
- Ironbark Honey

- Jarrah Honey
- Leatherwood Honey
- Linden Honey
- Macadamia Honey
- Manuka Honey
- Orangeblossom Honey
- Pinetree Honey
- Sourwood Honey
- Sage Honey
- Tupelo Honey

2. **Acacia Honey** Acacia is one of the most popular honey varieties. Identified as light and clear honey, it takes it delicate floral taste from the nectar of the blossoms of Robinia pseudo acacia, also known as Black Locust in North America and Europe. The high concentration of fructose helps acacia honey to retain its liquid state for a long period of time. Its low sucrose content makes it widely popular among the diabetics and with as a rich source of anti-inflammatory properties, it is best suited to treat respiratory disorders.
3. **Alfalfa Honey** Alfalfa honey is majorly produced in Canada and the United States. Made from the purple or blue blossoms, it is light in color and has a mild floral aroma and taste. Alfalfa Honey Due to its sweet yet mild taste, Alfalfa honey is often used for baking purposes. Though honey-enthusiasts prefer eating it straight out of the jar, it works better when combined with other ingredients like tea, lemonade and milkshakes among others.
4. **Aster Honey** This light-colored honey is majorly extracted from the Mid-South region of the United States. Aster Honey has a thick and smooth consistency accompanied by a distinctively sweet smell. It tends to crystallize faster than most other variety of Honey available and tastes best when used as a natural sweeter in a variety of sweet drinks and desserts.

5. **Avocado Honey** Avocado Honey doesn't taste anything like the fruit, but is extracted from the California avocado blossoms. It is a dark colored honey with a rich and buttery flavor and makes for a tasty salad dressing or condiment when mixed with other ingredients.
6. **Basswood Honey** Basswood Honey is most popular for its biting taste, distinctive white color and exceptional malleability quality that makes teaming it with any food item an easy job. Basswood Honey is produced from the cream-colored Basswood blossoms found throughout North America. It's fresh, pleasant and wood-like essence tastes incredibly well with a variety of teas and is hugely recommended for salad dressings and marinades.
7. **Beechwood Honey** Popularly known as Honeydew honey, it is sourced from New Zealand's South Island. It comes from the sap produced by aphids on the bark of the Beechwood tree and later collected by the bees. Beechwood Honey is widely used as syrup for pancakes and fruit salads due to its aromatic properties.
8. **Beechwood Honey** Its regular consumption is also known to improve the body's immunity, better the digestive system and is often used as a popular supplement due to its high nutritional value.
9. **Blueberry Honey** A pleasant flavor variety produced in New England and in Michigan, Blueberry honey is extracted from the white flowers of the blueberry bush. Light amber colored, a well-rounded flavor and a hint of tanginess from the Blueberry. Blueberry Honey makes for an ideal accompaniment for your breakfast meals like oats, pancakes and cereal bars.

10. **Bluegum Honey** This eucalyptus honey specie majorly grows in South Australia and Tasmania. Its dense texture and amber-color makes it a go-to topping for toasts and wafers. 8) Bluegum Honey's taste comes quite close to that of a bubble gum with a subtly cool and a minty undertone beneath its real dense texture.

11. **Buckwheat Honey** The strongest and darkest of honey varieties, Buckwheat Honey is mostly produced in Minnesota, Ohio, and Pennsylvania as well as in few eastern regions of Canada. As a rich source of iron and other essential nutrients,

Buckwheat Honey is among the most popular and widely consumed varieties of honey.

12. **Buckwheat Honey** It contains more antioxidant compounds than some lighter varieties of Honey in the same category.

13. **Clover Honey** Clover Honey is one of the most widely available and popular honey varieties in the world. It is majorly produced across Canada and New Zealand. Clover honey has been termed as a classic because of its pleasant and floral sweet taste, making it a hit ingredient for a vast variety of sauces and salad dressings.

14. **Dandelion Honey** Dandelion Honey is a relatively stronger variety of honey with mild blends of sourness in it. It is widely produced in New Zealand's South Island and is usually dark-amber in color. Dandelion Honey bears a characteristic Dandelion aroma, which is considered as a medicinal herb in China, Tibet and India due to its healing properties.

15. **Eucalyptus Honey** Originally originated in Australia, Eucalyptus Honey is widely extracted in California as well. A Great medicinal honey variety, Eucalyptus is traditionally used by people across the globe for protection against cold and headaches. Due to its extensive availability, Eucalyptus Honey differs in taste and flavor but carries a characteristic herbal flavor and a slight aftertaste of menthol.

16. **Fireweed Honey** Fireweed Honey comes from a tall herb grown in the open woods of north-west US. Light in color, it has its own way of being sweet and complex at the same time. Its smooth, delicate and buttery taste makes it a great option for gourmet cooking, baking and fish smoking.

17. **Heather Honey** One of the strongest and most pungent flavors available, Heather's aftertaste talks about being almost bitter and is commonly used as a spread or marinating Ham, chicken, lamb, seafood and cold meat dishes. Heather Honey is thick and amber in color and is known to be a rich source of protein.

18. **Ironbark Honey** Another premium Eucalyptus floral variety (Eucalyptus crebra) with a bold taste, Iron Bark Honey is

extracted from the blossoms throughout the year in eastern Australia. A favorite flavor catalyst for baking and barbecued meats, Ironbark Honey's amber color and dense texture adds a decadent taste to smoothies as well as other sweet drinks and shakes.

19. **Jarrah Honey** Jarrah is a dark- amber eucalyptus variety of honey that has a caramel aftertaste. Jarrah Honey has been scientifically researched to find out that Jarrah is an effective remedy for wounds, burns and skin allergies due to the higher percentage of activity level than most of the honey variety available in the market.

20. **Leatherwood Honey** Leatherwood Honey comes from the Leatherwood blossom in the south-west region of Tasmania, Australia. Leatherwood Honey is known for its unique taste and strong flavor. Also, commonly known as Tasmanian Honey, it has established itself as an irreplaceable ingredient that not only sweetens but also adds an excellent flavor to cakes, muffins, coffee and tea.

21. **Linden Honey** Light yellow in colour, Linden Honey bears a very delicate and fresh woody scent. One of the most medicinally rich varieties of honey, Linden has been a favorite for many before bedtime. Its sedative properties help immensely in the cases of anxiety and insomnia. Linden Honey is also used in the treatment of cold, cough and bronchitis. Extracted from Linden tree, which bears small yellowish white flowers, Linden honey is majorly produced in Denmark.

22. **Macadamia Honey** Macadamia Honey was first sourced in Australia from the floral nectar of the Macadamia Nut tree. It is deep in colour with a complex aroma and has a subtle nutty flavour. Macadamia Honey works well with salads, ice- cream, toasts and even as marinate for grilled chicken wings.

23. **Manuka Honey** Native to New Zealand's coastal areas, Manuka Honey is collected from the flower of the Tea Tree bush. It comprises of rich antibacterial property that aids in effectively treating stomach ulcers, sore throat, cold, indigestion and acne & pimples among others. Manuka Honey's taste varies due to the difference in source but usually boasts of a robust aftertaste that

stays for a while.

24. **Orangeblossom Honey** Orangeblossom Honey, often a combination of citrus sources, is usually light in colour and mild in flavour with a fresh fruity scent, and a fragrant citrusy taste. Originally originated from Spain/ Mexico, today Orangeblossom Honey is being produced in many countries including Florida, Southern California and Texas among others.

25. **Pinetree Honey** Pinetree Honey or Honeydew mainly comes from Greece. Quite opposite to the usual sweet taste of honey, Pinetree Honey has a slightly bitter taste with a strong aroma and is very rich in minerals and proteins.

26. **Sourwood Honey** Sourwood Honey is light-colored, delicate honey variety of Honey with a caramel kind of taste. While many find its taste to be sour, its hardcore followers find it to be as sweet and nutty as any other variety of Honey available.

27. **Sage Honey** The light-colored and heavy-bodied Sage Honey is mostly produced in California. Sage Honey is packed with a property to granulate very slowly and is commonly used to blend with other honeys to slow down the process of granulation.

28. **Sage Honey** Its mild yet delightful taste also makes it hugely popular with the consumers.

29. **Tupelo Honey** One of the most premium honeys ever produced, Tupelo Honey or the "Southern Gold", as it is popularly known as, is produced in the Southeastern U.S. swamps. It is usually light golden or amber in color with a faint greenish glow and a mild & distinctive taste. Tupelo honey is one of the sweetest honey varieties, courtesy the high fructose content and its ability of not granulating like most other types of Honey.

BENEFIT OF HONEY

1. Honey Contains Some Nutrients

Honey is a sweet, thick liquid made by honeybees. The bees collect sugar — mainly the sugar-rich nectar of flowers — from their environment. Once inside the beehive, they repeatedly consume, digest and regurgitate the nectar. The end product is honey, a liquid that serves as stored food for bees. The smell, color and taste depend on the types of flowers visited. Nutritionally, 1 tablespoon of honey (21 grams) contains 64 calories and 17 grams of sugar, including fructose, glucose, maltose and sucrose. It contains virtually no fiber, fat or protein It also contains trace amounts — less than 1% of the RDI — of several vitamins and minerals, but you would have to eat many pounds to fulfill your daily requirements. Where honey shines is in its content of bioactive plant compounds and antioxidants. Darker types tend to be even higher in these compounds than lighter types.

SUMMARY Honey is thick, sweet liquid made by honeybees. It is low in vitamins and minerals but may be high in some plant compounds.

2. High-Quality Honey Is Rich in Antioxidants

High-quality honey contains many important antioxidants. These include organic acids and phenolic compounds like flavonoids. Scientists believe that the combination of these compounds gives honey its antioxidant power. Interestingly, two studies have shown that buckwheat honey increases the antioxidant value of your blood. Antioxidants have been linked to reduced risk of heart attacks, strokes and some types of cancer. They may also promote eye health.

SUMMARY Honey contains a number of antioxidants, including phenolic compounds like flavonoids.

3. Honey Is "Less Bad" Than Sugar for Diabetics

The evidence on honey and diabetes is mixed. On one hand, it can reduce several risk factors for heart disease common in people with type 2 diabetes. For example, it may lower “bad” LDL cholesterol, triglycerides and inflammation while raising “good” HDL cholesterol. However, some studies have found that it can also increase blood sugar levels — just not as much as refined sugar. While honey may be slightly better than refined sugar for people with diabetes, it should still be consumed with caution. In fact, people with diabetes may do best by minimizing all high-carb foods. Keep in mind, too, that certain types of honey may be adulterated with plain syrup. Although honey adulteration is illegal in most countries, it remains a widespread problem.

SUMMARY Some studies show that honey improves heart disease risk factors in people with diabetes. However, it also raises blood sugar levels — so it cannot be considered healthy for people with diabetes.

4. The Antioxidants in It Can Help Lower Blood Pressure

Blood pressure is an important risk factor for heart disease, and honey may help lower it. This is because it contains antioxidant compounds that have been linked to lower blood pressure. Studies in both rats and humans have shown modest reductions in blood pressure from consuming honey.

SUMMARY Eating honey may lead to modest reductions in blood pressure, an important risk factor for heart disease.

5. Honey Also Helps Improve Cholesterol

High LDL cholesterol levels is a strong risk factor for heart disease. This type of cholesterol plays a major role in atherosclerosis, the fatty buildup in your arteries that can lead to heart attacks and strokes.

Interestingly, several studies show that honey may improve your cholesterol levels. It reduces total and “bad” LDL cholesterol while significantly raising “good” HDL cholesterol For example, one study in 55 patients compared honey to table sugar and found that honey caused a 5.8% reduction in LDL and a 3.3% increase in HDL cholesterol. It also led to modest weight loss of 1.3%.

SUMMARY Honey seems to have a positive effect on cholesterol levels. It leads to modest reductions in total and "bad" LDL cholesterol while raising "good" HDL cholesterol.

6. Honey Can Lower Triglycerides

Elevated blood triglycerides are another risk factor for heart disease. They are also associated with insulin resistance, a major driver of type 2 diabetes. Triglyceride levels tend to increase on a diet high in sugar and refined carbs.

Interestingly, multiple studies have linked regular honey consumption with lower triglyceride levels, especially when it is used to replace sugar. For example, one study comparing honey and sugar found 11–19% lower triglyceride levels in the honey group.

SUMMARY Elevated triglycerides are a risk factor for heart disease and type 2 diabetes. Several studies show that honey can lower triglyceride levels, especially when used as a sugar substitute.

7. The Antioxidants in It Are Linked to Other Beneficial Effects on Heart Health

Again, honey is a rich source of phenols and other antioxidant compounds. Many of these have been linked to a reduced risk of heart disease. They may help the arteries in your heart dilate, increasing blood flow to your heart. They may also help prevent blood clot formation, which can lead to heart attacks and strokes.

Furthermore, one study in rats showed that honey protected the heart from oxidative stress. All told, there is no long-term human study available on honey and heart health. Take these results with a grain of salt.

SUMMARY The antioxidants in honey have been linked to beneficial effects on heart health, including increased blood flow to your heart and a reduced risk of blood clot formation.

8. Honey Promotes Burn and Wound Healing

Topical honey treatment has been used to heal wounds and burns since ancient Egypt and is still common today. A review of 26 studies on honey and wound care found honey most effective at healing partial-thickness burns and wounds that have become infected after surgery. Honey is also an effective treatment for diabetic foot ulcers, which are serious complications that can lead to amputation. One study reported a 43.3% success rate with honey as a wound treatment. In another study, topical honey healed a whopping 97% of patients' diabetic ulcers. Researchers believe that honey's healing powers come from its antibacterial and anti-inflammatory effects as well as its ability to nourish surrounding tissue. What's more, it can help treat other skin conditions, including psoriasis and herpes lesions. Manuka honey is considered especially effective for treating burn wound.

SUMMARY When applied to the skin, honey can be part of an effective treatment plan for burns, wounds and many other skin conditions. It is particularly effective for diabetic foot ulcers.

9. Honey Can Help Suppress Coughs in Children

Coughing is a common problem for children with upper respiratory infections. These infections can affect sleep and quality of life for both children and parents. However, mainstream medications for cough are not always effective and can have side effects. Interestingly, honey may be a better choice, and evidence indicates it is very effective. One study found that honey worked better than two common cough medications. Another study found that it reduced cough symptoms and improved sleep more than cough medication. Nevertheless, honey should never be given to children under one year of age due to the risk for botulism.

SUMMARY For children over one year of age, honey can act as a natural and safe cough suppressant. Some studies show that it is even more effective than cough medicine.

10. It's Delicious, But Still High in Calories and Sugar

Honey is a delicious, healthier alternative to sugar. Make sure to choose a high-quality brand, because some lower-quality ones may be mixed with syrup. Keep in mind that honey should only be consumed in moderation, as it is still high in calories and sugar. The benefits of honey are most pronounced when it is replacing another, unhealthier sweetener. At the end of the day, honey is simply a "less bad" sweetener than sugar and high-fructose corn syrup

HONEY FOR WEIGHT MANAGEMENT

Honey can be very useful when you're trying to manage weight. Weight management* is one of the main benefits of honey! If you're overweight, honey not only helps you reduce weight but also reduces the risk of cardiovascular disorders.

Alright, hold on for us, in light of the fact that we couldn't trust it when we heard it either. Be that as it may, as indicated by new research, you could drop as much as a dress size in 3 weeks just by eating a spoonful of honey before bed each night.

By what means can something that is sweet and sugary help towards getting in shape, we hear you cry? Won't the calories in honey counter your efforts towards weight management? , it's all down to the metabolic force of honey. Honey triggers changes to the digestion system that guarantees you won't succumb to those troublesome sugar yearnings we all fall foul of and it even blazes fat while you rest!

Now you might wonder can diabetics eat honey. Worry not because compared to sugar, honey has more nutrients and vitamins along with more water content. But as it is said, anything in excess is always harmful. So people with diabetes can consume honey in moderation.

HOW CAN YOU USE HONEY FOR WEIGHT MANAGEMENT?

- Supplant Sugar with Honey
- Pick Unrefined Carbs
- Protein, protein, protein
- Follow the Hibernation Diet

1. **Improves Digestion** Disregard starving yourself and costly wellbeing nourishments - take after these straightforward principles and you could lose a few kgs in a week! Why not stick them on your refrigerator to offer you some assistance with remembering?
2. **Supplant Sugar with Honey** Cut out all sugar, including sweeteners, by using honey as an alternative. Start your day with honey in hot water, replace sugar with honey in tea and coffee, on cereal, and in all your cooking throughout the day. How will this help, we hear you ask? Let us help you understand better. Normal table sugar which is present in all of our houses contains calories which benefit you in absolutely no way. These calories, which give you very little or no nutrition are known as "empty calories". Your body uses up essential nutrients just to dissolve this unnecessary fat. Because most of our important nutrients and vitamins get used up here, we tend to gain weight while ingesting either pure sugar or sugar in other forms. This is exactly why honey, being a good source of nutrients, when substituted for sugar helps in reducing weight.
3. **Pick Unrefined Carbs** The refined white flour found in white

pasta and white rice can cause blood sugar spikes. Whole meal bread, pasta and brown rice are fiber-rich, so they are good for your digestion, take longer for your body to process and keep you feeling fuller for longer. Make sure that the whole meal carbs make up less than a quarter of your meal, and fill your plate with protein and vegetables.

TIPS TO MANAGE WEIGHT WITH HONEY

By making sure you have protein in every meal, you will feel fuller for longer and avoid blood sugar spikes leading to cravings. Try to keep protein as lean as possible to keep the calories down, such as fish (not breaded or battered), chicken (no skin), pork (fat trimmed), beef (steak or 5% fat mince) or eggs.

1. **Follow the Hibernation Diet** The hibernation diet is basically a diet that teaches us how we can manage weight while sleeping. Sounds too good to be true? In this diet, all you need to do is have a spoonful of honey before hitting the bed at night. This technique makes use of our biology. The honey fuels our liver which in turn speeds up the fat burning metabolism. Just like the name of this diet suggests, you can manage weight while hibernating.
2. **Improves Digestion** Honey has also been known to improve the functioning of the digestive system. Eating a spoon or two of honey after dinner works wonders. Especially when you've had a large meal, having a spoon of honey helps in reducing the static weight accumulated in your digestive system.
3. **Honey and warm water** Drinking water with honey can help you manage weight. Honey being a natural sugar, not only provides a healthy source of calories but also helps keep your sugar cravings at bay. Drinking honey and lemon water doesn't guarantee overnight Weight management* but it definitely helps the cause over a period of time.
4. **Honey and Lemon Juice** It is commonly believed that drinking honey and lemon water on an empty stomach in the morning speeds up Weight management. The combination of drinking warm water with honey and a few drops of lemon juice is a very important part of many Weight management* programs. Both honey and lemon have their own individual health benefits, when

combined together they not only help in Weight management but also cleanse your system of unnecessary fats.

5. **To make the honey- lemon drink:**

- Boil a glass of water and let it cool until it's warm.
- Add 2-3 spoons of Dabur Honey. Stir well till it dissolves.
- Squeeze 1/2 a lemon into this mixture.
- Stir this drink well and drink up.

6. **Honey and Cinnamon** You can also try our recipe of mixing cinnamon in honey and warm water to lose weight. We know this recipe sounds a bit bizarre but when honey and cinnamon are combined, they help you manage weight by reducing sweet cravings. Cinnamon has been known to stabilize the sugar levels in our blood. This prevents unnecessary storage of fat. Combine this with the benefits of honey and this recipe will have a positive impact on

your goal of Weight management.

WHILE USING HONEY FOR WEIGHT MANAGEMENT:

• Do not mix honey in boiling water

• Do not cook honey at high temperatures

• Doing any of the above mentioned acts will result in loss of nutrients because of the improper heat applied to honey.

• While following any diet, drill one thing in your mind: Not eating will not help you manage weight. Eating right will!

A diet doesn't always mean you have to starve yourself. Not eating enough food will definitely weaken your immune system as tonnes of calories, minerals and fibre will get accumulated in your system with no juice to burn it. Not eating when on a diet will only take you farther away from your goal of losing weight.

TRYING HONEY FOR WEIGHT LOSS

When a person is on a weight loss spree, he or she tries everything, from diet to workouts. Spending hours in the gym, cutting down on calories and so much more, but there's one thing which not many people try and that is honey and cinnamon water. Surprisingly, this simple mixture has amazing weight loss benefits. It helps you lose weight the easier way; and the best part is that it helps you melt belly fat first. Belly fat, which is linked to an increased risk of heart diseases, diabetes and some forms of cancer, is not easy to get rid of. But with honey and cinnamon you need not worry about that belly fat. Consuming honey right before bed time can help you burn more calories during the early hours of sleep. This ingredient is enriched with essential vitamins, minerals and healthy fats as well. Essential hormones in honey suppress appetite and aid weight loss.

Cinnamon, on the other hand, helps you lose visceral fat and supports weight loss. Antimicrobial, antiparasitic properties of cinnamon make it one of the healthiest spices of all time. It helps lower blood pressure, cholesterol, boosts insulin function and metabolism as well.

HONEY NUTRITION

Honey is quite useful in a lot of other things as well.

Honey Makes Excellent Cough The World Health Organization (WHO) lists honey as a demulcent, a substance that relieves irritation in your mouth or throat by forming a protective film. Research shows honey works as well as a dextromethorphan a common ingredient in over the counter cough medications, to soothe cough and related sleeping difficulties due to upper respiratory tract infections in children.

Honey Can Treat Wounds Honey was a conventional therapy in fighting infection up until the early 20th century, at which time its use slowly vanished with the advent of penicillin. Now the use of honey in wound care is regaining popularity, as researchers are determining exactly how honey can help fight serious skin infections.

Honey Improves Your Scalp Honey diluted with a bit of warm water was shown to significantly improve seborrheic dermatitis, which is a scalp condition that causes dandruff and itching. There was marked relief from itching and the scaling disappeared within one week. Skin lesions were healed and disappeared completely within 2 weeks.

Help Boost Your Energy A healthy, whole-food diet and proper sleep are the best recipe for boundless energy, but if you're looking for a quick energy boost, such as before or after a workout, honey does the trick.

Reduce Allergy Symptoms

Honey contains pollen spores picked up by the bees from local plants which introduces a small amount of allergen into your system. This helps activate your immune system and over time can build up your natural immunity against it.

Here's how you can prepare the honey and cinnamon water mix for weight loss:

1. Boil a cup of water and add half a teaspoon of cinnamon to it

2. Allow it to boil to 5 minutes

3. Remove it from the flame and allow it to cool

4. Once the drink cools down to room temperature, add one teaspoon of honey to it

5. Stir the drink properly and drink it

To make the most of the benefits of this weight loss drink, you need to drink it at the right time. Take note.

1. One cup of this weight loss drink before going to bed can prevent those late-night hunger pangs.

2. Drink this between the meals to curb your cravings your unhealthy junk foods.

3. Honey and cinnamon water is a great pre-workout drink, can help you stay energized during your workout sessions and can allow you to burn more fat as well.

4. One cup of this drink before and between your meals can save you from snacking after having your meals.

EXERCISE TO MANAGE WEIGHT

Let's admit it, every time we talk about wanting to manage weight, it's more about losing the inches of flab than about the numbers showing on the weighing machine. And most women have certain problem areas like the tummy, waist, hips, thighs or the butt etc. And that is the reason we tackle these areas specifically in the exercise tips below. Combine these exercises with the Honey Diet for a toned and fit body.

EXERCISE FOR THE STOMACH: SWAN DIVE

Get over the crunches and try this less stressful but equally effective exercise. Lie on your stomach and stretch your arms ahead while pointing your toes. Now, lift your arms and legs about 6 inches off the ground. Hold for 1 count, imagining your legs being pulled out and back, away from your hips. Next, circle your arms out to the sides and behind you. Exhale and reach your arms toward your toes, palms facing in. Hold for 1 count, then bring arms back to starting position and relax entire body to ground. Repeat 6–8 times.

EXERCISE FOR THE WAIST: THE ‘HUNDRED' EXERCISE

You can reduce the size of your waist by lying on your back and lifting your legs up to a 90 degree angle and your shoulder blades off the floor. Begin by pumping your arms straight out to the side and repeat for 100 pumps. Breathe in through the nose for five pumps and out through the mouth for five pumps. PS: This exercise is great for abs as well.

EXERCISE FOR THIGHS: STANDING SIDE KICK

Stand with your legs apart & hands on your hips and slowly extend your right leg to the side at hip height in 3 full counts. Ensure that you keep the inner thigh parallel to the floor. Now, hold for 1 count and then take 3 counts to lower to floor. Do this 15 times and then switch sides.

EXERCISE FOR HIPS: STAR JUMP

This exercise is high on energy and so it also helps to burn a lot of calories. Begin in a standing position with your feet together and arms at your sides. Slowly lower yourself into a squat and move your hands in front of your shins. Now, quickly jump off the floor and move your arms and legs out to your sides in an "X" pattern. Before you land, move your arms and legs back in. Lower yourself back down immediately and repeat.

EXERCISE FOR THE BUTT: WARRIOR

Who doesn't like a nice, toned butt? Try the Warrior exercise to look sexy in skirts and dresses. Stand with your feet together and lift your left leg with a pointed toe, putting your body weight onto the standing, right leg. Continue to lift your leg and drop the head & torso so they form a straight horizontal line from head to toe with the arms at your sides. Now, engage your core and make sure the left thigh, hip and the toes are aligned. Remain facing down and keep your back as straight as possible. Ensure your right knee doesn't lock and focus the weight on the middle of the foot. Hold for 5 breaths and then slowly return to standing. Now, switch legs and repeat.

DETAILING

Including honey diet in your daily routine can do wonders. Start your day with a hot toast and honey, or mix it in your tea (instead of sugar) and give your day a refreshing energetic start. You can also have a spoon of honey before you head out to your daily workout session, just to be able to go that extra mile, to lose that extra pound! Consuming honey in a drink, sandwiches and more can help your kids stay energetic throughout the day. No more lethargy for your children, or you. It would also interest you to know that a spoonful of honey before you sleep works wonders on your recovery cycle. Honey works excellently to reduce cholesterol levels. Fasting on honey and lemon juice is considered beneficial to battle obesity. It is so, because honey mobilizes extra deposited fat, and the body utilizes it as energy. Honey is your best friend, especially if you are a foodie! A spoonful of this tasty golden liquid after a heavy and oily meal will do wonders for your digestive system. It also works as a great detox tonic to keep your system healthy.

In all, consuming honey regularly helps improve your immunity system. Goodness of Honey works as a remedy for multiple ailments as well. Most of us know about the beauty benefits of honey, but did you know that honey is an effective ingredient for weight loss? According to research, you could drop a dress size in about three weeks, simply by taking a spoonful of honey before bed. Sounds too good to be true? Here's why honey works well for weight loss.

WHAT IS THE HONEY DIET?

Athletes who ate foods rich in fructose such as honey burnt a lot more fats and had increased stamina levels as well. Honey acts as a fuel to make the liver produce glucose. This glucose keeps the brain sugar levels high and forces it to release fat burning hormones. To benefit from the honey diet, simply replace your sugar intake with honey, throughout the day. In addition to that you should consume three spoonfuls of honey with hot water every night before bed. Combine this with an exercise regime (try and exercise three times a week) and you will notice a sizeable drop in your weight.

The study showed that the mechanism in the brain that caused the sugar craving could be shut down completely with this honey routine.

HOW IT WORKS?

Most of us struggle to lose weight because we consume too much sugar and processed food. When we consume honey before bed, the body begins to burn more fat during those early hours of sleep. When you go a step further and replace all refined sugar from your diet with honey, you rebalance the brain signal that compels you to consume more sweet stuff. The results noticed from the honey diet have been remarkable. But remember to keep these points in mind: Replace all sugar with honey: Cut out sugar from your diet. This means you will also have to give up on artificial sweeteners. Use honey in your tea, coffee and cereal instead of refined sugar. Keep a check on what you cook too, so that you don't use sugar in there either. Skip junk food: Junk foods are processed food that contains empty calories. To fully benefit from the honey diet, stop eating junk food. Opt for unrefined carbs: Refined white flour in white pasta and white rice may cause a spike in blood sugar levels. Opt for wholemeal flour instead as they are good for digestion and will keep you fuller for a longer time.

Consume Proteins: Keep your proteins lean but make sure you consume proteins with every meal as it will keep you full and also avoid a blood sugar rise that leads to cravings. Be careful with your fruits: Fruits are a convenient option while dieting but remember that most fruits are high in sugar levels and can hamper your honey diet. Either reduce your fruit intake or opt for low-carb fruits like berries and rhubarb. No potatoes: Any form of potato can cause your body's insulin level to rise. The honey diet requires you to avoid eating potatoes.

HONEY AND WEIGHT LOSS-WHATS THE SCORE

As part of an overall calorie-controlled diet, and as a replacement for refined sugar, honey can play it's part in a diet, in small quantities. For example, if you allow yourself a spoon of sugar in your tea as part of your overall diet regime, you could substitute sugar for honey instead. However, whether or not it really makes a significant difference, I'm not so sure. One thing is for certain: honey is a high energy food, so it is unlikely to help you lose weight when consumed in excess - quite the opposite, and I can't imagine lots of honey would be very helpful for your teeth either! As with all things; too much of a good thing....can turn into a bad thing.

CONCLUSION

Know your BMI and ideal body weight to help set your goals and track your progress. Your ultimate goal at a minimum should be to get your BMI in the normal range and an aggressive goal would be to get down to your ideal body weight. Understand the concept of calories and how they relate and sometimes do not relate to weight loss and weight gain. Know your basal metabolic rate (BMR) and % body fat to track your progress. Know the total number of calories you burn in a day (BMR + daily activity + exercise), but do not worry much about how many calories you eat as long as you stick to a whole foods plant based diet to achieve this goal. An aggressive weight loss goal is to lose 2 pounds per week. So if we were counting calories as the only factor (which they are not) we would say each pound is 3500 calories, your body needs to use 7000 more calories per week than you eat. With 7 days in a week, that means you need to burn off 1000 more calories per day than you eat.

A more realistic goal is 1 pound per week, which is 3500 per week or a 500 calorie deficit per day. The guidelines from the ACC/AHA/TOS recommend a 500-750 calorie deficit per day for safe weight loss. They specifically recommend a 5-10% reduction in weight in the first 6 months, which will usually come out to 1-2 pounds per week. Just focus on eating healthy foods such as fruits, vegetables, beans/legumes, whole grains, and nuts/seeds and counting calories will be completely unnecessary

www.ingramcontent.com/pod-product-compliance
Lightning Source LLC
LaVergne TN
LVHW090135160826
845673LV00017B/2477

9798474773483